USMLE STEP 2 CK
Cardiology
In Your Pocket

✓ Study guide for the USMLE STEP 2 CK exam.

✓ Prepare for your shelf examination.

✓ Be ready for your inpatient rotation.

.

Gregory J. Fernandez M.D.

First Edition, 2016

Author & Editor: Gregory J. Fernandez, M.D.

Publisher: M.D. Educational Services

Peer-reviewers: Urshilkumar Patel, M.D. & Rajat Eshan Lamington, M.D.

Book Design: Marie Meyer

Copyediting: Editage Cactus Communications

DISCLAIMER: The author, editor, publisher, and staff members have taken care to confirm the accuracy of the information present in this publication. The context of the books entirety, is believed to be reliable in accordance with the standards accepted at the time of publication. However, readers are encouraged to confirm the information and conduct their own research for clarification of all the information present within this book. No one involved in creating this book is responsible for errors or omissions or for any consequences from application of the information in this book. There is no warranty, expressed or implied, with respect to the completeness or accuracy of the contents of this publication. Neither the editor, nor the author assumes any liability for any injury and/or damage to persons or property arising from the content of this publication. Application of this information in a particular situation remains the professional responsibility of the practitioner; the clinical treatments or information described and recommended may not be considered absolute and universal recommendations. It is the responsibility of the health care provider to ascertain the FDA status of each drug used or device planned for use in their clinical practice. The purpose of this books, is to be used as a study guide for medical examinations. Please consult with attending physicians for any medical decisions.

ISBN-13: 978-1530481873

ISBN-10: 1530481872

This book is gratefully dedicated to my wife. Thank you for your support and always being there for me. Thank you for your kindness, your devotion, and your endless selflessness support. I love you… Thank you mother, father, step-mother, brothers, friends, and family for all your encouragement and endless love. Best of luck to all the medical dreamers, the road is long and I hope my book helps you through this journey. All the best…

How to Use
"Cardiology In Your Pocket"

Cardiology In Your Pocket is a study guide for the USMLE STEP 2 CK exam that you can also use to prepare for your shelf examination and to get ready for your inpatient rotation. It is part of a series, each dealing with a different subject or sub-specialty, focusing on vital clinical knowledge.

The subjects and topics within cardiology are called out in large, colored type. These items are also included in the Table of Contents for ease of access.

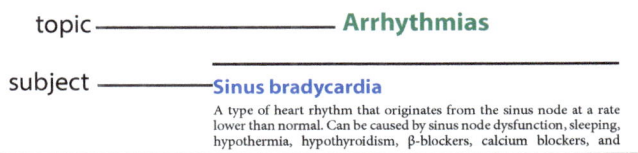

Many subjects also contain sub-subjects that are called out in bold, blue type, either as bulleted items or in-line with the text, as appropriate. They are all referenced in the index.

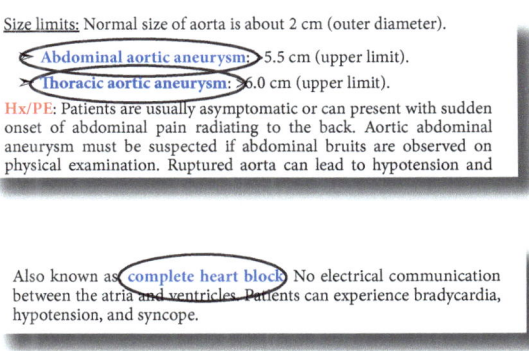

Presentation of clinical history and physical exam (Hx/PE), step-by-step diagnosis, and treatment plan are indicated by bold red headings.

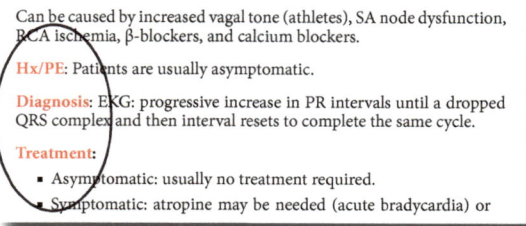

Can be caused by increased vagal tone (athletes), SA node dysfunction, RCA ischemia, β-blockers, and calcium blockers.

Hx/PE: Patients are usually asymptomatic.

Diagnosis: EKG: progressive increase in PR intervals until a dropped QRS complex and then interval resets to complete the same cycle.

Treatment:
- Asymptomatic: usually no treatment required.
- Symptomatic: atropine may be needed (acute bradycardia) or

Procedures, triads, pathology, medications, antibodies and findings are called out in bold text. These items are also included in the index.

- IV fluid expansion (also apply to right-sided infarct).
- Urgent **pericardiocentesis** (needle drainage), especially in unstable patient.
- In case of severe or long-term condition **cardiac window** needs to be considered.
- If stable and secondary to uremic pericarditis, then consider dialysis.

Reflexes, signs and maneuvers are shown in purple text.

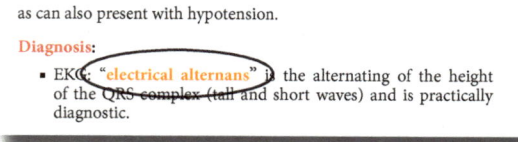

Hx/PE: **Becks triad**: hypotension, JVD, and decreased heart sounds. Patient present with tachycardia and tachypnea. Pulsus paradoxus (decrease in systolic blood pressure >10 mmHg with normal inspiration). Need to rule out dehydration and pulmonary embolism; as can also present with hypotension.

Mnemonics and key words are shown in orange text.

as can also present with hypotension.

Diagnosis:
- EKG: "electrical alternans" is the alternating of the height of the QRS complex (tall and short waves) and is practically diagnostic.

And, finally, for the avoidance of doubt, circumstances that amount to a medical emergency are flagged with a warning.

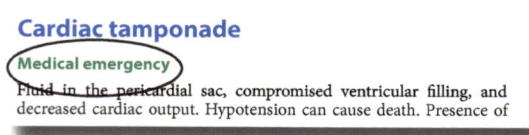

Cardiac tamponade
Medical emergency
Fluid in the pericardial sac, compromised ventricular filling, and decreased cardiac output. Hypotension can cause death. Presence of

Cardiology
Table of Contents

cont'd on next page

Cardiology
Table of Contents, cont'd

Arrhythmias

Sinus bradycardia

A type of heart rhythm that originates from the sinus node at a rate lower than normal. Can be caused by sinus node dysfunction, sleeping, hypothermia, hypothyroidism, β-blockers, calcium blockers, and athletes (marathon runners).

Hx/PE: SOB (*most common* symptom), chest pain, hypotension, and syncope.

Diagnosis:

- EKG: <60 bpm with sinus rhythm (defined as P-wave before QRS complex).
- Review medications and check TSH, glucose, electrolytes, and toxicology.

Treatment:

- *Asymptomatic*: no treatment.
- *Symptomatic*: atropine (*first line*) or epinephrine and treat underlying pathology.
- No response to atropine and symptomatic, place temporary pacemaker.
- *Long-term treatment:* pacemaker (*most effective*).
- If hypotensive: administer IV fluids and/or atropine if no signs of fluid overload.

Note: placement of a permanent pacemaker might be needed for long-term treatment for sinus bradycardia, and stabilization with transcutaneous pacing will be needed prior to the surgery.

Sinus tachycardia

A heart rhythm that is produced in the sinoatrial (SA) node, which produces a heart rate higher than normal. It can be either normal physiological tachycardia or abnormal pathological tachycardia.

Risk factors: fear, pain, anxiety, hypoxia, anemia, pulmonary embolism, hypoglycemia, asthma, hyperthyroidism, dehydration, medications, and exercise.

Hx/PE: SOB, lightheadedness, palpitations, chest pain, and rapid pulse.

Diagnosis:

- EKG: sinus rhythm (P-wave before QRS complex) at >100 bpm.
- Labs based on suspicion:
  - Basic labs: CBC, electrolytes, TSH, glucose levels, urine toxicology, and pulse oxygen.

Note: quick estimate of heart rate on EKG is by counting each large box from QRS complex to QRS complex (300, 150, 100, 75, 65, 50, and 30).

Treatment:

- Often asymptomatic and requires no treatment (normal physiological tachycardia).
- Treatments for underlying pathological causes, which may include: administration of β-blockers, calcium blockers, IV fluids, pain-relief medication, oxygen, transfusion, etc.

First-degree atrioventricular (AV) block

Results in a prolonged PR interval >200ms. First-degree AV block can be caused by a disease in the electrical conducting system (AV node), increased vagal tone (athletes), myocardial infarctions, β-blockers, and calcium blockers.

Hx/PE: Patients are usually asymptomatic.

Diagnosis: EKG: prolonged PR interval of >200 ms or 0.20 seconds.

Treatment: No treatment necessary. Discontinue problematic medications and treat underlying myocardial infarctions.

Note: EKG do not always reveal arrhythmias and will need a 24-hour Holter monitor for further investigation.

Second-degree block, Mobitz Type I (Wenckebach)

Can be caused by increased vagal tone (athletes), SA node dysfunction, RCA ischemia, β-blockers, and calcium blockers.

Hx/PE: Patients are usually asymptomatic.

Diagnosis: EKG: progressive increase in PR intervals until a dropped QRS complex and then interval resets to complete the same cycle.

Treatment:

- *Asymptomatic*: usually no treatment required.
- *Symptomatic*: atropine may be needed (acute bradycardia) or consider pacemaker.

Second-degree block, Mobitz Type II

Associated with fibrotic disease, AV node dysfunction, His-Purkinje system dysfunction, or prior myocardial infarction. Has a high risk of developing a third-degree block.

Diagnosis: EKG: two P-waves for every one QRS complex.

Treatment:

- Consult cardiology for pacemaker placement even if asymptomatic.
  - *First*, place a transcutaneous pacemaker.
  - *Next*, place a transvenous pacemaker.

Third-degree block

Also known as, complete heart block. No electrical communication between the atria and ventricles. Patients can experience bradycardia, hypotension, and syncope.

Diagnosis: EKG: no relationship between the P-wave and QRS complex.

- In *acute* cases of syncope, atropine can be used.
- Consult cardiology for pacemaker placement:
  - *First*, place a <u>transcutaneous</u> pacemaker.
  - *Next*, place a <u>transvenous</u> pacemaker.

Atrial fibrillation

A rapid irregular arrhythmia that is usually from an ectopic source. They can be caused by myocardial ischemia, mitral stenosis, hypertension, hyperthyroidism (sympathetic activity), chronic heart failure (CHF), ASD, sepsis, rheumatic fever, pulmonary disease, or ethanol. Patients are at high risk of clot formations (DVT).

Hx/PE: Palpations, chest pain, SOB, and irregular pulse.

Diagnosis:

- EKG: "**irregular irregular**" QRS (erratic) and possible "**F-waves**."
- If fibrillation cannot be detected on EKG, then 24-hour Holter monitoring will be required.
- All patients should be screened for hyperthyroidism (TSH and FT4).
- Order general labs: CBC, electrolytes, glucose levels, TSH, troponins (if chest pain), urine toxicology, and chest x-ray.

Treatment:

- *First step*: rate control with medications (β-blockers or calcium blockers).
  - Metoprolol or esmolol (β-blockers) or diltiazem (calcium blocker).
- *If stable*: common medications are "**ABCD**" <u>a</u>nti-coagulation (if fibrillation lasts for more than 48 hours), <u>β</u>-blockers, <u>c</u>alcium-blockers, or <u>d</u>igoxin. Anticoagulants must be administered if the condition lasts for more than 2 days.
- *Unstable* or *new onset*: synchronized cardioversion is recommended for patients who are hemodynamically unstable:

- If chest pain, dyspnea, hypotension, or confusion is observed, shock should be delivered to the patient.

Note: in cases of hypotension, COPD, or asthma, its best to administer calcium blockers, as β-blockers can exacerbate these symptoms.

Atrial flutter

An abnormally regular heart rhythm caused by a re-entrant impulses occurring in the atria of the heart.

Hx/PE: Syncope, SOB, chest pain, and palpations.

Diagnosis:

- EKG: heart rate (atrial >300 bpm), "**sawtooth appearance**," and smooth P-waves (look the same).
- Symptomatic or undiagnosed palpitations require 24-hour Holter monitoring.
- Order: CBC, electrolytes, TSH, glucose levels, urine toxicology, troponins, chest x-ray, and echocardiogram.

Treatment:

- *Stable*: "**ABCD**" <u>a</u>nti-coagulation, <u>β</u>-blocker, <u>c</u>alcium blocker, and <u>d</u>igoxin.
    - *First stabilization of patient* followed by anticoagulants.
- *Unstable*: synchronized cardioversion (in case of chest pain, SOB, hypotension, or confusion).

Note: β-blocker contraindications must be taken into consideration.

Multifocal atrial tachycardia

An abnormal rhythm, arising from multiple ectopic foci within the atria. Associated with COPD and emphysema. Most commonly occurs with lung disease but can occur from low potassium, low magnesium, CHF, and post MI.

Hx/PE: SOB, dizziness, chest pain, and palpations.

Diagnosis: EKG (heart rate >100 bpm and at least three different P-wave formations from the same EKG lead) or 24 Holter monitor.

Treatment: Oxygen, replacement of potassium and magnesium, and either calcium blockers or beta-blockers (controversial).

Note: use beta-blockers with caution as most of these patients have COPD.

Premature ventricular contractions (PVCs)

Is a premature beat from an ectopic source arising from the ventricular foci (purkinje fibers). Causes include hypoxia, medications, alcohol, electrolyte imbalance, and hyperthyroidism.

Hx/PE: Palpitations or asymptomatic, SOB, and syncope.

Diagnosis:

- EKG: <u>wide</u> QRS complex not preceded by P-waves. If unsure use 24-Holter monitoring.
- Check for underlying causes such as electrolytes, TSH, and ABG.

Treatment:

- *Asymptomatic*: treat underlying cause (hypoxia or electrolytes). Correct magnesium, calcium, and potassium.
- *Symptomatic*: administer β-blockers.

Premature atrial contractions (PACs)

Cardiac dysrhythmia that results in premature beats arising from the atria. This condition can be caused by caffine intake, alcohol consumption, stress, and smoking. May lead into atrial flutter or atrial fibrillations.

Hx/PE: Palpations or often asymptomatic, syncope, and SOB.

Diagnosis:

- EKG: often normal findings.
- If patient is symptomatic, 24–72-hour Holter monitoring will be required.

Treatment:

- *Asymptomatic*: no treatment other than reassurance; avoid consumption of alcohol, coffee, and smoking.
- *Symptomatic*: administer β-blockers.

Ventricular tachycardia

An abnormal heart rate arising from abnormal electrical conduction of the ventricles of the heart. Common with coronary artery disease (CAD).

Hx/PE: Syncope, palpation, SOB, and chest pain.

Diagnosis:

- 12-lead EKG: beats are regular, rapid, and demonstrate <u>wide</u> QRS complex.
    - Wide QRS complex tachycardia and no distinct P or T waves, is presumed to be ventricular tachycardia until proven otherwise.
- When a diagnosis is not possible by EKG, then place patient on telemetry monitoring.
- Order: CBC, electrolytes, TSH, glucose, and toxicology.

Treatment:

- *Stable*: amiodarone, lidocaine, or procainamide (*better choice* than lidocaine).
- *Unstable*: synchronized cardioversion.
- **Pulseless ventricular tachycardia**:
    - The *first* step is shock (<u>un</u>synchronized cardioversion);
    - If no response, *then* give epinephrine;
    - If no response, *then* deliver shock again;
    - If no response, *then* give amiodarone.

Note: synchronized defibrilator (200J) can be done if identifiable QRS complex or in patients who have a pulse. A defibrillator automatically determines if the QRS complex is present.

Ventricular fibrillation

Described as uncontrolled ventricular contractions, which can be a common arrhythmia that occurs during cardiac arrest or sudden death. Can rarely be reversed spontaneously. It is commonly associated with CAD and myocardial infarction.

Hx/PE: Absence of blood pressure and pulselessness.

Diagnosis: EKG (erratic wide-complex tracing).

Treatment:

- Immediate defibrillation (unsynchronized) is *the most important step.*
- Unsynchronized cardioversion is the *first step*, even before intubation.
- After defibrillation, follow the ACL protocol without interruption.

Note:

- ✓ A hemodynamically unstable patient will require cardioversion, regardless of the type of cardiac arrhythmia.
- ✓ Unsynchronous cardioversion is used for pulseless ventricular tachycardia, ventricular fibrillation, and Torsades de pointes.

Torsades de pointes

Prolonged QT-interval that can be congenital or acquired; often caused by abnormal electrolytes, malnourished, and common in alcoholic patients.

Hx/PE: Palpation, dizziness, and syncope.

Diagnosis: EKG: polymorphous QRS, varying from beat-to-beat "twisting" around the isoelectric line.

Treatment:

- *Stable*: IV magnesium sulfate (*first-line treatment* and prevention).
  - Can infuse despite magnesium baseline.

- If magnesium sulfate infusion has no effect, consider temporary pacemaker placement.
- Treat hypokalemia, hypocalcemia, and hypomagnesemia.

- *Unstable*: immediate, <u>un</u>synchronized cardioversion.

Supraventricular tachycardia (SVT)

Characterized by a rapid regular rhythm causing a circle like re-entry of current around the P-wave.

Diagnosis: EKG: regular rhythm heart rate of >180 bpm, <u>narrow</u> QRS, and abnormal or absent P-waves (no P-wave).

Treatment:

- *Stable*: *first step* is carotid massage, Valsalva maneuver, or immersion of the face in ice water (to help <u>decrease</u> AV node conduction).
    - If the initial measures do not control SVT, *first-line treatment* is IV **adenosine** therapy.
    - *Secondary medications* (usually administered after three attempts with adenosine): β-blockers or calcium blockers.
- *Unstable*: synchronized DC cardioversion (SOB, chest pain, confusion, and hypotension).
- *Best long-term treatment* is radiofrequency catheter ablation.

Note: carotid massage should <u>not</u> be given, in case of carotid bruit (carotid stenosis).

Wolf-Parkinson-White syndrome

Congenital accessory conduction pathway between the atrium and ventricle, and rapid conduction down the *accessory pathway*.

Diagnosis: EKG: short PR intervals (<0.12 seconds), wide QRS, followed by slow depolarization through the ventricle leading to a "delta wave."

Treatment:

- *If stable*: *best initial* treatment is **procainamide**.
- *If unstable*: synchronized cardioversion (rule of thumb is to deliver shock in case of SOB, chest pain, hypotension, or confusion).
- *Best long-term treatment* is catheter-ablation therapy.

Note: a side effect of procainamide is drug-induced SLE.

Pulseless electrical activity (PEA)

A feature of clinical cardiac arrest where no pulses are detected on physical examination, however, EKG demonstrates electrical production. PEA has an abnormal response of the cardiac tissue to the electrical impulse. Technically, there should be a pulse but no pulse found on palpation.

Hx/PE: No pulses found on physical examination (best places for pulse palpation are the femoral artery and carotid artery).

Diagnosis: EKG: commonly shows disorganized electrical activity or sinus rhythm.

Treatment:

- *First choice* is cardiopulmonary resuscitation (CPR) with chest compressions and epinephrine (vasopressor) 1 mg every 3 - 5 minutes.
- Atropine is not recommended for PEA or asystole.

Note: defibrillation or cardioversion is not a component of resuscitation for PEA, as the problem is abnormal response of the cardiac tissue to the electrical impulse.

Asystole

Asystole is different from pulseless electrical activity because asystole has no electrical activity and therefore, no cardiac tissue response. Patients show no pulse or electrical activity. Asystole can be used to confirm legal death.

Diagnosis: EKG (no electrical activity).

Treatment: Epinephrine 1 mg every 3 - 5 minutes as needed in combination with CPR.

Note: asystole is <u>not</u> a shockable rhythm (a defibrillator cannot detect the QRS complex and deliver shock). Here again, atropine is not used for asystole.

NYHA - CHF

<u>Class I:</u> no limitation, and no symptoms with activity.

<u>Class II</u>: mild limitation only with activity.

<u>Class III</u>: moderate discomfort with activity.

<u>Class IV</u>: discomfort at rest.

Note: CHADS score:

- ✓ **C** = CHF (1 point).
- ✓ **H** = Hypertension (1 point).
- ✓ **A** = Age > 75 years (1 point).
- ✓ **D** = Diabetes (1 point).
- ✓ **S** = Stroke or TIA (1 point for each)
  - If CHADS score is 0–1, give aspirin.
  - If CHADS score is >2, give warfarin.

Note: more current recommendations, is use of the **CHA2DS2-VASc score** over the original CHADS2 score to assess stroke risk in patients with atrial fibrillation.

Cardiomyopathies

Systolic dysfunction

Decompensated heart failure with insufficient contractions, which leads to decreased ejection fraction, increased preload, increased afterload, increased left ventricular workload, and CHF.

Hx/PE: Orthopnea, nocturnal dyspnea, chronic dry cough, and lower extremity edema (bilateral).

Diagnosis:

- Diagnosis initially obtained by history and physical examination.
- Electrolytes: hyponatremia (none specific but can determine severity).
- The water retention of systolic dysfunction causes hyponatremia.
- EKG: low-voltage QRS complex.
- Chest radiography: cardiomegaly, cephalization of pulmonary vessels, pleural effusions, and blunting of costophrenic angles bilaterally (represents CHF).
- Optimal initial test is echocardiogram: decreased ejection fraction and left ventricular dilation.
- Multiple gated acquisition scan (MUGA): non-invasive and *accurate* method to determine EF.
- Brain natriuretic peptide (BNP) level > 500 pg/mL (usually checked to *confirm* diagnosis).

Treatment:

- In cases of *acute* fluid overload and SOB, administer IV furosemide (for symptomatic relief).
- *Long-term acute treatment*: control comorbidities, limit salt and fluid intake, add ACEIs/ARBs and β-blockers (if not decompensated CHF).
    - Both ACEIs and β-blockers *decrease mortality.*
- Digoxin is used for *long-term therapy* for CHF with decreased ejection fraction <u>but</u> dobutamine is more useful in *acute exacerbation* of CHF.

- Pulmonary edema: use furosemide and nitrates.
  - If not resolved, use dobutamine (a positive inotrope) to decrease afterload; it can cause hypotension, which can be treated by dopamine.
- Spironolactone is used in late stages of CHF to inhibit aldosterone levels, but can cause gynecomastia and hyperkalemia.
- When dilated cardiomyopathy is observed with an ejection fraction <35 and QRS above 120 ms, use a biventricular pacemaker.

Note: CHF increases GFR, renin, aldosterone, and fluid levels, which can lead to hyponatremia.

Other considerations:

- ASA and statins help prevent ischemic heart disease.
- Loop diuretics (furosemide) decrease fluid overload.
- Pulmonary edema: consider furosemide, oxygen, nitrates, and morphine.
- Embolic events or atrial fibrillation: consider warfarin.
- Digoxin relieves symptoms but does not decrease mortality (measure electrolyte levels before administering).

Fun facts:

- Transfusions can exacerbate CHF.
- *Most common* risk factor for CHF is CAD.
- CHF needs to be treated before any major surgery.
- *Most common* cause of death of CHF are arrhythmias.
- The *most accurate test* for determining the ejection fraction is MUGA scan (precise evaluation of wall motion abnormalities).
- Transesophageal echocardiogram (TEE) is not necessary for evaluation of CHF but is an optimal method for evaluating the valves.
- Diuretics and digoxin do <u>not</u> decrease mortality.
- Spironolactone regulates the functioning of the renin-angiotensin aldosterone system and <u>decreases</u> mortality by decreasing the fluid load and exertion of the heart in CHF patients.

- Low levels of potassium increases digoxin toxicity.

- ACEIs elevates potassium levels and therefore, decrease digoxin toxicity.

- A CHADS score of zero can be managed without anticoagulants or aspirin.

- A CHADS score of >2 should be managed with anticoagulation therapy.

Note: mortality benefits: ACEIs/ARBs, β-blockers, spironolactone, nitrates, hydralazine, and implantable defibrillator. Warfarin can be used in patients with a low ejection fraction to decrease mortality.

Dilated cardiomyopathy

A condition where the heart is enlarged and cannot pump blood effectively, which causes systolic dysfunction, decreased ejection fraction, left ventricular dilation, increased afterload, and increased preload. The condition causes secondary constriction of the efferent arteriole leading to increased GFR (increased sodium and water retention) and exacerbated lower extremity edema (bilateral).

Hx/PE: Orthopnea (worsens when lying flat), nocturnal dyspnea, peripheral edema, rales, elevated jugular venous pressure, and S3 heart sounds.

➤ Primary causes: "ABC³D": alcohol consumption, beriberi disease, cocaine use, coxsackie virus infection, Chagas disease (protozoan are more common in Central and South America), and doxorubicin use.

➤ Secondary causes: CAD, hypertension, peripheral vascular disease (PVD), and CHF.

Diagnosis:

- Electrolytes: hyponatremia.

- EKG: low-voltage QRS and sinus tachycardia.

- ABG: respiratory alkalosis (SOB).

- Chest radiography: cardiomegaly (>50% of thoracic diameter), **Kerley B lines** (fluid between the lobes), and pleural effusions (blunting of the diaphragm).

- *Most important test*: echocardiogram (decreased ejection

fraction, left ventricular enlargement, and thin-walled ventricle).

- <u>PCWP</u> (elevated pressure in the left atrium).

Note: CHF work-up with echocardiogram (*most important test*) to determine whether patient has systolic dysfunction or diastolic dysfunction; severity can be measured by the ejection fraction, and then confirmed with BNP levels.

Treatment:

- Decrease intake of salt and fluids and add diuretics (furosemide).
- Mortality can be decreased by preventing cardiac remodeling with β-blockers (in cases of non-decompensated CHF or pulmonary edema), spironolactone, and ACEIs (EF <40%).
- Digoxin: in case of CHF with ejection fraction <35%, and pacemaker application should be considered.
- Pulmonary edema: medication considerations are oxygen, diuretics, nitrates, and morphine. These medications help decrease cardiac preload.

<u>Prevention</u>: exercise, diet, weight loss, smoking cessation, and alcohol cessation.

Note: use statins for high-risk patients even with borderline cholesterol levels.

Diastolic dysfunction

Diastolic dysfunction

An abnormality where the heart muscles do not relax in a normal manner, which affects how the heart fills with blood during diastole. Diastolic dysfunction is commonly caused by hypertension and CAD.

Hx/PE: SOB, chest pain, and lightheadedness.

Diagnosis:

- Physical examination: S4 gallop.
- EKG: left axis deviation.

- Chest x-ray: normal or slight cardiomegaly.
- Echocardiogram (increased ejection fraction) *gold standard.*

Note: increased ejection fraction, decreased ventricular compliance, and left ventricular hypertrophy.

Treatment:
- Control blood pressure with β-blockers (*first line*), as medication shows clear benefits.
- Calcium blockers (verapamil [nondihydropyridine]) and ACEIs may have a benefit mainly because of their action in decreasing cardiac remodeling.

Note: digoxin would never be used for diastolic dysfunction.

Hypertrophic cardiomyopathy (HCM) vs. hypertrophic obstructive cardiomyopathy (HOCM)

➤ **Primary (HOCM)**: AD, diastolic dysfunction, increased ejection fraction, hypertrophy of the left ventricle, sudden death in athletes, S4 murmur, systolic anterior motion, and "harsh midsystolic crescendo-decrescendo" murmur at the apex.

Hx/PE: SOB is the *most common* symptom. The murmurs for HOCM are different from most pathological murmurs:

  ➤ Increases intensity of the murmur: Valsalva maneuver, standing up, and administration of nitrates.
  ➤ Decreases intensity of the murmur: squatting, handgrip, lying down, and leg elevation.

➤ **Secondary (HCM)**: *most common* causes are hypertension, PVD, or aortic stenosis.

Hx/PE: SOB (dyspnea) is the most common symptom, followed by chest pain and lightheadedness.

Overall diagnosis:
- EKG: left ventricular axis and sinus tachycardia.

- Chest radiography: normal or slightly enlarged cardiac silhouette.
- Echocardiogram: left ventricular hypertrophy and increased ejection fraction.

- *Asymptomatic*: no treatment and most importantly avoid competitive sports for HOCM.
- *Symptomatic*: β-blockers (*first line*) or calcium blockers (*second line*).
- *Diuretics may be helpful in HCM but contraindicated in HOCM.
- If above treatments fail, **myomectomy** will relieve obstruction in the left ventricular outflow tract.

Note:

✓ Digoxin is never an appropriate treatment for HOCM or HCM.

✓ In both systolic and diastolic failure can administer β-blockers and ACEIs.

Side effects of digoxin: Hypokalemia, gynecomastia, gastrointestinal (GI) problems, and visual problems (yellow halos). If the toxicity levels increase, the drug should be stopped and K+ supplementation should be started, and **digoxin-binding antibody** (if CNS or cardiac problems) should be administered.

Restrictive cardiomyopathy

Restrictive cardiomyopathy

A rare disease of the myocardium with its principle abnormality being diastolic dysfunction (restricted ventricular filling) and decreased elasticity. Caused by amyloidosis, sarcoidosis, hemochromatosis, fibrosis, and scarring. The cardiac walls cannot relax or contract.

Hx/PE: Dyspnea (*most common* complaint), elevated JVD, edema, ascites, and organomegaly. Kussmaul sign (increase in JVD on inhalation).

Diagnosis:

- <u>EKG</u> (low-voltage QRS).
- <u>Chest radiography</u> (normal or calcifications present).
- <u>Echocardiogram</u> (*gold standard*) ejection fraction can be normal or elevated.
- *Most accurate test*: **endomyocardial biopsy** (fibrosis) rarely done.

Treatment:

- Treat underlying causes/palliative only.
  - Secondary to sarcoidosis (use steroids).
  - May require cardiac transplant.
- Diuretics (for fluid overload).
- Warfarin (for atrial fibrillation).

Coronary artery disease

Coronary artery disease (CAD)

Also known as **ischemic heart disease** and includes stable angina, unstable angina, and myocardial ischemia. CAD is the *most common* type of heart disease and the leading cause of death in the United States among both men and women.

Hx/PE: "**Dull chest pain radiating to the jaw or left arm**," palpitations, SOB, nausea, vomiting, and diaphoresis. Rarely, chest pain is exacerbated or alleviated with respiration. Diabetic and elderly patients may present with atypical symptoms (no chest pain).

*If pain changes with respiration, palpation, or position, the differential diagnosis needs to be broadened.

Diagnosis: EKG (*first test*), chest radiography, troponin levels (*most accurate test*), echocardiogram, stress test, and angiography.

Note: in cases of epigastric pain, perform immediate EKG.

<u>Rule out</u>: GERD (clinical diagnosis or 24-hour pH monitoring), pneumonia (chest radiography), costochondritis (physical

examination), angina (EKG and troponins), myocardial ischemia (EKG and troponins), and acute pancreatitis (lipase and abdominal CT scan).

Note: GERD is the *most common* cause of chest pain.

Treatment:

- Look below at "overall treatment of myocardial infarction" for more details.
- In a very clear case of ischemia, treatment can be administered before laboratory tests.
- Aspirin is always the *first choice* medication (timing is critical).
- β-blockers: decrease mortality and morbidity by decreasing the heart rate and blood pressure.
- ACEIs: help decrease blood pressure and risk of future heart attacks in patients with prior history.

Cholesterol prophylaxis: statin daily (morning).

Platelet prophylaxis: aspirin daily (81 mg).

Health prophylaxis: diet, exercise, weight loss, smoking cessation, and alcohol cessation.

Note:

- Smoking cessation provides immediate benefit and within 2 years of cessation, the risk of CAD reduces by 90%.
- *Single most* dangerous risk factor for CAD is diabetes.

Angina

Stable angina

Is mainly caused by CAD, which is an atherosclerotic disease obstructing the arteries that deliver blood to the heart. Symptoms such as, chest pain are precipitated by activity and relieved at rest.

Hx/PE: Chest pain with ambulation and relieved at rest. Pain is described as dull, heavy, and tight. "Dull pain" is a key term used to describe cardiac ischemia.

Diagnosis:

- *Best initial test*: EKG (decreased ST-segment) and <u>no</u> troponin level elevation.
- Stress test (exercise vs. drug-induced) results can be normal.
- In cases of <u>positive</u> stress test results, a coronary angiogram would be the *next step*.

Note: EKG findings for stable angina can be normal or abnormal during acute attacks or stress test.

Treatment:

- Symptoms are not present at rest and improve with nitroglycerin (relieves pain).
- *Most important long-term treatments*:
  - Diet, exercise, and weight loss.
  - Control of hypertension, DM, and hyperlipidemia.
  - Educate patient on smoking cessation and alcohol intake.
- Medication considerations: nitrates, aspirin, statins, and β-blockers.
- Surgical considerations: angioplasty, stenting, and bypass.

Fun facts:

- ACEIs are not recommended for treating stable angina.
- In patients with stable angina, angioplasty does not improve mortality only the symptoms.
- Chronic angina mortality is decreased with β-blockers and aspirin.
- Can differentiate stable angina from GERD, as GERD worsens with nitroglycerin.

Unstable angina

Unstable angina occurs at rest or with minimal exertion and usually lasts about 5 minutes.

Hx/PE: New onset of worsening symptoms (chest pain) and increased episodes even during rest.

Diagnosis:

- *Optimal initial test*: EKG (decreased ST-segment and no troponin level elevation.
- Obtain a stress test (exercise vs. drug induced). Results more likely to be abnormal as compared to those obtained from stable angina.
- In case of positive stress test result, a coronary angiogram must be obtained.

Treatment:

- Symptoms are present at rest and improve with nitroglycerin.
- "MONA-B" morphine, oxygen, nitrates, aspirin, and β-blockers.
- Treatment is similar to that administered for stable angina with addition of heparin and GPIIb/IIIa.
- Surgical considerations: angioplasty (also called percutaneous coronary intervention [PCI]), stenting, and bypass.

Long-term treatment: Exercise, weight loss, daily aspirin, statins, and diet.

Note: smoking cessation must be encouraged, alcohol intake should be limited to <4 Oz/day, and lifestyle modifications should be made (exercise and diet).

Prinzmetal's angina

Vasospasm of the coronary arteries that causes temporary narrowing of the arteries and transient ischemia. Can be caused by cocaine use, Raynaud phenomenon, or smoking.

Hx/PE: Chest pain is described as "spasmic-type pain."

Diagnosis:

- EKG: elevated ST-segment with no elevation of troponin levels.
- Stress test can also show normal results.
- *Most accurate test* for diagnosis is coronary angiogram to view the vasospasms (but can often show normal results).

Treatment: Calcium-channel blockers such as verapamil and nitroglycerin (relax coronary artery spasms).

Note:

✓ ST-elevations with elevated troponin level are more likely to be observed in STEMI than in Prinzmetal's angina.

✓ In *severe* cases of Prinzmetal's angina, troponin levels can be elevated.

Fun facts:

- Aspirin and β-blockers (can cause additional vasospasms) are <u>not</u> helpful.

- If vasospasm caused by cocaine use and accompanied with hypertension, consider benzodiazepines, IV nitroglycerin, or phentolamine.

Myocardial infarction

Non-ST-elevation myocardial infarction (NSTEMI)

Considered a <u>partial</u> obstruction of the blood vessels in the heart. This condition resembles unstable angina (depressed ST-segment) but with <u>elevated</u> troponin levels. It involves worsening of unstable angina and increase in troponin levels, indicating cardiac damage.

Diagnosis:

- EKG: non-elevated ST-segment with elevated troponin levels.
    - If chest pain has been present for many days or weeks, troponin levels might not be helpful.
    - Chest radiography: used to rule out other pathologies.
- If positive stress test results are obtained, coronary angiogram must be performed to decide whether the patient needs percutaneous coronary intervention (PCI) or CABG.

Treatment:

- *Acute symptoms*: "MONA-B" <u>m</u>orphine (used for pain and dilation of the blood vessels), <u>o</u>xygen, <u>n</u>itrates (dilation of capacitance vessels), <u>a</u>spirin (*first medication* given), and β-blockers (reduce oxygen demand of heart).

- Anticoagulant drugs prevent reinfarction and can be achieved by using unfractionated heparin or low molecular weight heparin.
- If stress test shows negative results, the patient can be discharged on "A²BC²" (aspirin, ACEIs, β-blockers, clopidogrel, and cholesterol-busting statins).

Prevention: diet, exercise, weight loss, smoking cessation, and alchol cessation.

ST-elevation myocardial infarction (STEMI)

A complete obstruction of the blood vessels of the heart. STEMI is a worsened NSTEMI that shows ST elevations and increased troponin levels; indicating a worsening ischemia. STEMI is worse than NSTEMI and demonstrates worse cardiac damage.

Diagnosis:

- Order: EKG (*first test*), chest radiography, and serial troponin levels (q6-hour).
    - EKG: elevated ST-segment and troponin levels.
- Elevation in anterior leads such as V2-V4 is associated with a worst prognosis.

Note: ST changes are the first to occur on an EKG.

Treatment:

- Similar to the *initial treatment* of NSTEMI: "MONA-B" should be given, if no contraindications.
- ST-elevations of >2 mm in at least two leads, will need to be treated with thrombolytics or PCI (if no contraindications).
- Aspirin should be given before thrombolytics.
- Aspirin plus clopidogrel decrease cardiovascular events more than just aspirin alone.

Long-term treatment: "A²BC²" (ASA 81 mg/d [lifelong], ACEIs, β-blockers, clopidogrel [6 to 12 months], and cholesterol busters [statins]). Control diet, exercise, weight, HTN, DM, and lipids.

Note: for STEMI use clot busters as clots have already formed (tPA is used to dissolve clots).

Overview of myocardial infarctions and angina

Common causes of chest pain

➤ Chest pain radiating to the back:
- Aortic dissection (*most accurate* test is a CT angiography) or pancreatitis (lipase and abdominal CT scan).

➤ Tracheal deviation:
- Pneumothorax (*most accurate* test is chest radiography).

➤ Cough, fever, and sputum production:
- Pneumonia(*first test* is chest radiography).

➤ Worsens when lying flat and improves when standing:
- Pericarditis (*most accurate* test is EKG [ST elevations in all leads]).

➤ Sudden onset of chest pain, SOB, tachycardia, hypoxia, and hypotension:
- Pulmonary embolism (*most accurate tests* are spiral CT scan, angiogram, and V/Q scan).

Complications of myocardial infarction

- *Ventricular fibrillation* (loss of pulse): common cause of death in the first 24 hours.

- *Septal rupture:* new murmur and oxygenation of the right side of the heart.

- *Free wall rupture:* can lead to cardiac tamponade, usually occurs about 3–5 days after MI.

- Avoid steroids after a myocardial infarction as they can cause ventricular wall rupture.

- *Valvular rupture:* new murmur.

- *Papillary muscle rupture:* needs to be corrected with surgery, which usually results in mitral valve regurgitation and can happen as soon as 12 hours after MI.

- *Right ventricular infarction:* lungs usually with clear breath sounds.

- *Tamponade/wall rupture:* increased JVD, hypotension, and decreased breath sounds.
- *Third-degree AV block* ("**cannon A**" waves): start atropine; pacemaker needed.
- *Compartment syndrome:* can also be caused by arterial occlusion.
- **Dressler's syndrome** (similar to pericarditis): is an autoimmune disease occurring within the cardiac tissue after an ischemia. It must be treated with high-dose aspirin, NSAIDs, or steroids.

Diagnosis of myocardial infarction
- EKG (*best initial test*): ST-segment elevation or depression of >2 mm (males) and >1.5 mm (females) in at least 2 leads is diagnostic of MI.
    - With ST elevation clots have already formed and non-ST-elevation clots are about to be formed.
    - Leads V1–V4 most likely due to occlusion of the left anterior descending artery (anterior).
    - Leads II, III, and AVF = Inferior MI (involves LCA, RCA, and PDA).
    - Leads V1–V2 = Posterior MI (PDA).
    - Leads I, AVL, V5–V6 = Lateral wall MI (LCA).
    - Normal axis: leads I (up) and II (up).
    - Left axis: leads I (up) and II (down).
    - Right axis: leads I (down) and II (up).
    - Symptomatic patients do not need to wait for cardiac marker results for treatment, if elevated ST segments on EKG.
- Chest radiography: rule out pneumonia, pulmonary edema, and aortic dissection.
- Myoglobin is a *non-specific* marker of heart damage; can be elevated in 1-2 hours post-MI (this is the *first* enzyme to be elevated after an MI).
- Troponins: cardiac enzymes that can have elevation within 3 hours of onset and remains present for at least 10 days. If troponin levels are negative before 3 hours, will need to re-measure.

- In case of suspected reinfection, <u>CPK-MB</u> (lasts for about 1-2 days), which has a shorter half-life than troponins.
- <u>Stress testing</u>: performed when other diagnostic tests fail to establish the diagnosis. An angiography is not needed, unless the stress test shows abnormal results.
    - The stress test is performed to detect abnormalities when other diagnostic tests do <u>not</u> yield positive results and there is high suspicion.
- <u>Angiography</u> is the *next best step* after an abnormal stress test.
- In cases of abnormal angiography results, surgical intervention must be considered.
- Echocardiography is the *best initial test* to evaluate abnormal valves and ejection fraction.

<u>Treatments for myocardial infarction</u>

- Medications that *lower mortality*: aspirin, β-blockers, clopidogrel, tPA, and PCI.
- ASA (325 mg) should be the *first* medication given in case of active ischemia to decrease mortality.
- Angioplasty has a greater potential of *lowering mortality* than tPA.
- Angioplasty has the *greatest mortality benefit*, but aspirin should still be given first (even before angioplasty).
- Angioplasty is associated with fewer hemorrhagic complications and is less likely to lead to development of new MI.
- ACEIs: mortality benefits are the highest when ejection fraction is <40%.
- All patients should be placed on statin medication after a baseline liver function test.

<u>Non-mortality benefits for myocardial infarction</u>

- Oxygen, nitroglycerin, and morphine are <u>not</u> associated with a clear mortality benefit.

<u>Overall treatements of myocardial infarction:</u>

- <u>Aspirin (325 mg):</u>
    - Always the first medication to be given (for mortality benefits). Works immediately and the timing is critical.

- **β-blockers** (mortality benefits):
    - While the timing is <u>not</u> as critical, they must be given as soon as possible, if there are no contraindications. The coronary arteries are filled during diastole. This is why β-blockers are so important, as they decrease heart rate.
- **ACEIs or ARBs:**
    - Should be given to all patients but are beneficial more in patients with systolic dysfunction, low EF, or CHF. These medications also have *mortality* benefits.
- **Calcium blockers:**
    - Used if intolerance to β-blockers, severe asthma, hypotension, or bradycardia.
    - Use in Prinzmetal's angina.
- **Amiodarone and lidocaine:**
    - Use in ventricular tachycardia or ventricular fibrillation (might have some benefit).
- **Nitrates::**
    - These provide pain relief but no mortality benefits.
- **Pacemaker:**
    - Use for third-degree AV block, Mobitz IIa (rarely), and Mobitz IIb.
- **Heparin:**
    - It prevents clot formation but does <u>not</u> dissolve clots that are already formed.
    - One of the most important first steps is IV heparin for NSTEMI.
- **Thrombolytics:**
    - *First*, consider FOBT to rule out active bleeding and rule out other contraindications.
    - tPA should be considered for STEMI (<u>not</u> NSTEMI).
    - New LBBB is also an indication of tPA.
    - tPA must be administered within 30 minutes of entering the hospital for mortality benefits. As time increases from dosage time, the mortality benefits decrease.
    - Can be beneficial for up to 12 hours but more beneficial if

given within 3 hours of onset.

- *Fibrin* (leads to clot formation) and *plasmin* (destroys the clots). tPA activates plasmin.
- Factor XIII (stabilizes clots) and tPA needs to be given <u>before</u> factor XIII stabilizes the clots.
- tPA acts as a clot buster as long as factor XIII has not formed.
- Thrombolytics have no benefit for NSTEMI, however, lower mortality if cases of ST elevations or new LBBB.
- If tPA is contraindicated then angioplasty (e.g., PCI) must be considered.
- Streptokinase should not be given rapidly, as this medication can cause allergies.

- <u>Angioplasty</u>:
  - PCI is a type of angioplasty.
  - Angioplasy is performed more often in STEMI than NSTEMI.
  - PCI is more effective than tPA for STEMI.
  - Needs to be performed within 90 minutes of entering the hospital.
  - Glycoprotein IIb/IIIa inhibitors: inhibit the aggregation of platelets and can be used in patients who undergo angioplasty and stenting.
    - Also, can be indicated for unstable angina or NSTEMI, or asprin allergy.
  - If a stent is used, clopidogrel plus aspirin are used to help keep blood vessels open.
  - Stent options: bare metal stent, drug-eluting stent (*best*), and no stent.
  - PCI complications: coronary artery rupture, restenosis, and hematoma at the entry site.

- <u>Statins</u>:
  - Should be given to all patients with hyperlipidemia, ACS, MI, angina, stroke, TIA, and PAD.
  - The *most common* adverse effect is liver toxicity, not rhabdomyolysis.

- Side effects of myocardial infarction medications:
  - Clopidogrel rarely causes TTP and neutropenia.
  - Clopidogrel is *more* effective as an antiplatelet medication than aspirin.
  - Ticlopidine (inhibits platelets) is rarely used and can cause neutropenia.
  - ACEIs can cause dry cough (switch to ARBs) and hyperkalemia.
    - Angioedema is rarely caused by ACEIs, if develops switch to ARBs (lower risk of angioedema).
  - Nitrates are contraindicated to use with sildenafil (can cause severe hypotension).
    - Can give IV fluids and epinephrine, if develops.
  - Beware of using β-blockers in cases of hypotension, bradycardia, COPD, severe asthma, or cardiogenic shock.
  - Most patients with moderate asthma can tolerate β-blockers.
  - Low molecular weight heparin (LMWH) is superior to unfractionated heparin in terms of mortality benefits.
  - Unfractionated heparin is preferred over LMWH in cases of renal failure.

EKG findings after myocardial infarction

- **RBBB**: causes include pulmonary hypertension, RVH, PE, pulmonary stenosis (note pathology is on the right heart).
- **LBBB**: causes include aortic stenosis, LVH, systemic hypertension (note pathology is on the left heart).

   Note: LBBB during ischemia caused by MI is worse than that caused by RBBB.

- **Paradoxical split**: the pulmonary valve closes <u>before</u> the aortic valve (normally the aortic valve should close before the pulmonary valve). Common in aortic stenosis.
- **Left circumflex coronary artery**: supplies the lateral wall of the left ventricle.
- **P-wave**: atrial depolarization, **QRS wave**: ventricular depolarization, and **T wave**: ventricular repolarization.

Physical examination for myocardial infarction patients:

- S4 sound is a sign of LVH.
- S3 sound is a sign of dilated left ventricle (sounds splashy on physical examination).
- If changes in position or touch alter the chest pain, it is most likely <u>not</u> ischemia.

Risk Factors and post-MI precautions

- Diabetic patients have the *highest* overall risk of myocardial infarction after 10 years of diabetic history.
- Women and men have the *same* risk of CAD after 65 years of age.
- Women in the reproductive age (< 55) rarely experience MI; need to look for other sources.
- Family history is positive if the father is <45 years or mother is <55 years of age experiencing first MI.

Post-myocardial infarction precautions:

- Sexual activity is recommended to resume about 4-6 weeks after an MI, if free of symptoms.
- Exercise can begin at about the same time, and the intensity can be gradually increased as tolerated.
- Weight loss is more likely to improve blood pressure than diet and exercise.
- The *single largest* risk factor for CAD is diabetes.
- Smoking cessation is the *most important* behavioral change for decreasing the risk of myocardial infarction.
- Exercise increases HDL levels and decreases LDL levels.
- Blood pressure for renal failure and diabetes patients should be maintained at <130/80 mmHg.
- Always keep in mind that diabetics and elderly patients can show atypical symptoms.
- ** SOB in a diabetic may warrant an EKG and troponin levels evaluation.
- SLE patients are at an increased risk of premature coronary atherosclerosis, and this is a common cause of death among these patients.

- After a myocardial infarction, the *best predictor* of prognosis is the ejection fraction.

Right ventricular infarct

Described as right ventricular failure caused mainly by an inferior wall myocardial infarction.

Hx/PE: Resembles cardiac tamponade on physical examination (hypotension, elevated JVD, and tachycardia). Can present with clear lung sounds.

Diagnosis:

- EKG: ST interval abnormalities in the lower leads (such as II, III, and AVF). Lead V1 is the *only* lead that truly looks directly at the right ventricular. However, the *most useful* lead is V4R, which can be evaluated by placing the V4 electrode in 5th right intercostal space midclavicular. In case of ST-elevation in V4R, 78% *specific* and 88% *sensitivity*. ST elevation in V1 and ST depression in V2 is also *specific* for right ventricular infarct.

Treatment:

- IV fluids (*first-line treatment)* to keep preload high.
- Consider thrombolytics, angioplasty, antiplatelet, aspirin, and statins.
- *Contraindications* for right ventricular infarct: nitrates, morphine, or diuretics. Also, use beta-blockers and calcium blockers with caution.

Note: right ventricular infarct should <u>not</u> receive medications that decrease preload, such as nitrates, morphine, or diuretics. If these medications are given, give IV bolus of isotonic saline to optimize right ventricular preload.

Stress test

Exercise stress test

A stress test is a way to measure the hearts ability to external stress in a controlled environment. Test helps diagnosis CAD, prognosis post-MI, identify abnormal heart rhythms, and exercise tolerance levels.

- Conducted stress test when diagnosis is <u>not</u> clear (normal resting EKG findings and normal troponin levels) and when ischemic disease is highly suspected.

- In high risk patients consider coronary angiogram before exercise stress test.

- Never conduct stress test when patient has active chest pain (contraindicated).

- Stress test results are positive when there are <u>ST-depressions</u> of >1 mm that last longer than 0.08 seconds.

- If the stress test results are <u>positive</u>, the *next step* is to perform a **coronary angiogram** (*most accurate* method to detect CAD) for assessing the need for possible revascularization.

    - If the coronary angiogram shows 1–2 vessels disease, use angioplasty. **Angioplasty** involves opening of the vessels by ballooning and holding vessels open often with stent placement.

    - If the coronary angiogram shows 2–3 vessels disease, perform coronary artery bypass grafting (CABG).

- **CABG** indicated if:

    - Significant left main coronary stenosis, with >50% stenosis.

    - Severe proximal LAD, with >70% stenosis and EF <50%.

    - Proximal left circumflex artery, with >70% stenosis.

    - 3-vessel disease, with >50% stenosis.

    - 2-vessel disease, in patients with diabetes.

- If the stress test result after MI is negative, the *next step* is to discharge the patient on aspirin, clopidogrel, β-blockers, ACEIs, and statins.

- Also, discharge patient with sublingual nitrates, as needed for acute chest pain.
- If the patient given standard treatment and chest pain persists, catheterization will be needed.

Note:

- ✓ Stress testing should be performed <u>only</u> after MI has been excluded with serial negative troponins.
- ✓ These interventions (angioplasty and CABG) pose a risk of systemic cholesterol embolization (**blue toe syndrome**).
- ✓ If the stress test result is negative, discharge the patient.
- ✓ If the stress test result is positive, then further intervention will be delivered.
- ✓ Do not cause ST-elevations during the stress test, as this would be like creating an actual MI.

Exercise thallium test

The stress test can be conducted with adenosine or dobutamine.

- If the patient has no contraindications or baseline abnormalities, perform exercise treadmill stress test instead of exercise thallium test.
- Exercise thallium test is performed if the EKG has baseline abnormalities or patient has arthritis, exercise intolerance, pacemaker, LBBB, digoxin use, obesity, claudication, lower extremity ulcer, dementia, amputation, or WPW.
- Stress echocardiogram is more sensitive than stress EKG.

Note:

- ✓ Adenosine is contraindicated in COPD and asthma, as this medication can cause bronchospasm.
- ✓ If the patient has asthma, use dobutamine.

Submaximal stress test

- Test performed 5–7 days <u>after</u> an ischemic attack.
- 70% of the target heart rate is sufficient (target heart rate = 220 – age).

Maximal stress test

- Test performed 2–3 weeks <u>after</u> an ischemic attack.
- 80% of the target heart rate is sufficient (target heart rate = 220 – age).

Vascular pathologies

Abdominal aortic aneurysm (AAA)

This condition occurs when the abdominal aorta artery enlarges by >50% of its diameter or about 3 cm.

<u>Risk factors</u>: smoking (*#1 risk factor*), hypertension, atherosclerosis, hyperlipidemia, and vascular disease.

<u>Size limits:</u> Normal size of aorta is about 2 cm (outer diameter).

➤ **Abdominal aortic aneurysm**: >5.5 cm (upper limit).

➤ **Thoracic aortic aneurysm**: >6.0 cm (upper limit).

Hx/PE: Patients are usually asymptomatic or can present with sudden onset of abdominal pain radiating to the back. Aortic abdominal aneurysm must be suspected if abdominal bruits are observed on physical examination. Ruptured aorta can lead to hypotension and abdominal pain.

Diagnosis:

- On physical examination, listen for abdominal bruits.
- *Initial test of choice* is abdominal ultrasound (use for diagnosis and follow-up).
- If asymptomatic and size is less than size limits, monitor with an abdominal ultrasound every 6–12 months.
- Abdominal CT scan (used for *precise* anatomy for surgery).
- In case of rupture, surgery must be conducted <u>before</u> radiological studies.

Note: abdominal ultrasound might not be useful for obese patients. If obese patient, abdominal CT scan will be more helpful.

Treatment:

- *Asymptomatic patients*: the most important step is blood pressure control and smoking cessation.

  - Asymptomatic patients must be monitored with abdominal ultrasound.

- *Symptomatic patients*: surgical intervention will be necessary.

- **Emergency surgery** is necessary if the aneurysm is rapidly growing, ruptured, or above the size limit.

Screening: Men should be screened with a single screening abdominal ultrasonography if >65 years of age and a history of smoking.

Note: a few days after AAA surgery there is a risk of ischemic colitis that will necessitate a colonoscopy to monitor signs of ischemia and necrosis.

Aortic dissections

Medical emergency

Blood between the aortic layers secondary to a tear in the *tunica intima*, usually <u>above</u> the aortic valve and distal to the left subclavian artery. The *number one* risk factors is hypertension and trauma. The leading cause of death in patients with Marfan's syndrome.

Hx/PE: Sudden "**ripping pain**" radiating to the back, asymmetric pulses in the upper extremities, new aortic regurgitation (early diastolic), and crescendo-decrescendo murmur.

Pain relationship (nonspecific):

- ➤ If the pain is radiating to the anterior chest, <u>ascending</u> dissection must be considered.

- ➤ If pain is radiating to the back, <u>descending</u> dissection must be considered.

Diagnosis:

- The *first step* is to manage blood pressure with IV medications before studies.

- The *optimal initial diagnostic test* is chest radiography (widening of the mediastinum or aortic knob).

- TEE: can be done at bedside, especially if patient presents with renal failure.
- *Most accurate test* is spiral CT scan or CT angiography.

Treatment:

- *Most important step* is to control blood pressure with IV β-blockers. If <u>not</u> controlled with β-blockers can consider vasodilators (sodium nitroprusside).
- Esmolol is a good choice in acute setting, as it has a *short half-life*. Labetlol is also commonly used.
- <u>Ascending dissection:</u> emergency surgery after blood pressure control.
- <u>Descending dissection:</u> *first* manage blood pressure and heart rate (*first choice medication* is labetalol). In complicated cases need to also consider surgery.

Note: systolic blood pressure should be maintained to the lowest tolerable levels.

Hypercholesterolemia

Hypercholesterolemia

Cholesterol level >200, LDL level >130, HDL level <40, and triglycerides level >500.

<u>Risk factors</u>: poor diet, lack of exercise, OCPs, nephrotic syndrome, diabetes, family history, obesity, hypertension, hypothyroidism, Cushing's syndrome, and thiazide use.

- ➤ **Xanthomas**: nodules on the skin and tendons.
- ➤ **Xanthelasmas**: yellow fatty deposits around the eye.

Diagnosis:

- Elevated fasting lipid profile (at least 8 hours of fasting) on 2 occasions.
- Rule out hypertension, DM, and other underlying factors.

- *First step* is 12-week trial of diet, exercise, and weight loss (if stable and no risk factors).
    - Diet and exercise need to be encouraged to lower LDL level to <160 (if no risk factors).
- If unsuccessful, start medication (statins are most commonly used).
- Treat all patients with medications with LDL levels ≥190.
- Refer to the endocrinology section of *In Your Pocket* for more details.

Start screening lipid levels at the age of 35 years for men and 45 years for women.

Note:

✓ If statin toxicity (CPK levels >10x upper limits of normal) then discontinue until CPK normalizes.

✓ Tests that require fasting are lipid testing, glucose testing, and hydrogen breath test (lactose deficiency).

Hypertension

Primary (essential) hypertension

No identifiable cause and observed in 95% of hypertension patients. Hypertension is a risk factor for atherosclerotic disease and is the *most important* modifiable risk factor for stroke.

Risk factors: obesity, smoking, alcohol, family history, race, gender, age, high salt diet, and African American ethnicity.

Diagnosis:

- Diagnosed with blood pressure of >140/90 mmHg on two separate occasions at least 1 week apart.
- 24-hour blood pressure monitoring (*most accurate method*).
- In case of *severe hypertension* or stage 3 hypertension (>180/110 mmHg), treat immediately (IV anti-hypertensive medications).

- Newly diagnosed hypertension needs work-up for CBC, electrolytes, urinalysis, fasting glucose levels, EKG, and fasting lipid profile.
- Always perform eye examination (fundoscopy), renal examination (BUN/Cr ratio and microalbuminuria), peripheral examination (pin-prick), abdominal examination (bruits), and carotid artery examination (bruits).
- Aging adults will usually present with increased systolic pressure, decreased diastolic pressure, and increased pulse pressure.

Note: need to monitor brain (stroke/hemorrhage), eye (cotton-wool/hemorrhage), kidney (proteinuria), PVD, and posterior nose bleeding.

Treatment:

- **Prehypertension** (120-139/80-89 mmHg).

  -If no risk factors, control with diet and exercise.

  -No treatment unless end-organ damage (renal disease) or other comorbidities (DMI or DMII).

- **Stage 1 hypertension** (140–159/90–99 mmHg).

  - Benefits of treatment for stage 1 hypertension is controversial.

  - Can try diet and exercise for 3 months, and if not controlled, add a thiazide only if there are   no other comorbidities.

  - ACEs or ARBs and β-blockers in case of comorbidities or specific conditions:

  > CAD: use β-blockers.

  > Osteoporosis: use thiazide.

  > Pregnancy: use α-blockers.

  > Depression, asthma, or COPD: do not use β-blockers.

  > BPH: use α-blockers.

  > Hyperthyroidism: use β-blockers.

  > Diabetes: use ACEIs or ARBs.

  > Migraine: use β- blockers or calcium blockers.

  > CHF: use β-blockers, ACEIs, or ARBs.

- **Stage 2 hypertension** (160–179/100–109 mmHg).

Need a two drug combination regiment, always use ACEIs with β-blockers (unless contraindicated). There are several medical combinations that can be used.

Note:

✓ **Isolated systolic hypertension** (common in elderly population): Systolic pressure >160 mmHg and diastolic pressure <90 mmHg. Use calcium blockers as a mode of treatment (to lower mortality rate).

✓ Calcium blockers are also effective for hypertension in African-Americans (as this population can show resistance to β-blockers).

Note: causes of **secondary hypertension** such as, hyperthyroidism, congenital adrenal hypoplasia, thyroid dysfunction, Conn syndrome, pheochromocytoma, renal failure, and others (which are covered in other sections).

Hypertensive urgency

Hypertension with only mild to moderate symptoms <u>without</u> end-organ damage.

Diagnosis: These are a few laboratory results and findings to consider urinalysis (microalbumin level), troponin level, EKG, LFTs, head CT-scan findings, and ophthalmic examination findings.

Treatment:

- Use <u>oral</u> medications: β-blockers, clonidine, or ACEIs.
- Lower blood pressure over 24–48 hours.

Hypertensive encephalopathy

Sever hypertension causing mental status changes.

Hx/PE: Headache, restlessness, AMS, seizures, and papilledema.

Diagnosis: Head CT scan without contrast (ischemia vs. hemorrhage), EEG, EKG, troponin level, urinalysis, and eye examination.

Treatment: IV nitroglycerin (*fast and short half-life*) or <u>IV</u> labetalol. Once blood pressure is controlled switch to oral medications.

Hypertensive emergency

Severe hypertension with impending end-organ damage.

Diagnosis: Need to monitor organs: troponins, EKG, chest x-ray, LFTs, urine microalbumin, BUN/Cr ratio, and optic examination.

Treatment:

- Use IV medications: nitroprusside (*best acute* IV medication). Remember, it can be harder to control the blood pressure response elicited by sublingual nitrates than by IV medications.
- IV labetalol (beware of asthma, bradycardia, and AV block).
- Hydralazine (mainly administered to pregnant patients and children) can lead to reflex tachycardia.
- Nicardipine.

Note: no more than 25% decrease in blood pressure over the first 2 hours to prevent cerebral hypoperfusion and coronary insufficiency.

Malignant hypertension

Medical emergency

Hypertension with progressive renal failure and/or encephalopathy with papilledema (specific finding). Pailledema must be present before a diagnosis of malignant hypertension is made.

Hx/PE: Headache, restlessness, AMS, seizures, and papilledema.

Diagnosis:

Treatment <u>before</u> diagnostic testing.

- CBC, electrolytes, BUN/Cr ratio, urinalysis, LFTs, troponins, EKG, head CT scan, and chest x-ray.
- Rule out blood alchol levels and urine toxicology
- Evaluation of patients will depend on their symptoms and your medical judgment):
  - If papilledema, performing an ophthalmic examination.
  - If focal findings, head CT scan might be the *first* evaluation test.

- *First step* is to decrease blood pressure (IV medications such as nitrates or labetalol) and then perform evaluation tests.
- Patient will need cardiorespiratory monitoring.

OCP-related hypertension

Might cause a slight elevation in blood pressure in about 5% of women. More common among women who are aged >35 years, obese, and on long-term OCP use. Also, consider hyperlipidemia with OCPs.

Treatment: *First step* is to discontinue OCPs.

A few important anti-hypertensive medications

Hydrochlorothiazide (HCTZ)

Mechanism: reduces sodium reabsorption in the distal convoluted tubules.

Usage:

- *First-choice* diuretic for patients with stage 1 hypertension (with no other risk factors).
- Administered to patients with osteoporosis (increases re-uptake of calcium).
- Used in case of nephrolithiasis (calcium oxalate stones), as it helps reabsorb calcium.
- Used to treat diabetes insipidus.

Side effects:

- "GLUC": elevated glucose, lipids, uric acid, and calcium levels.
- Allergies to sulfa medications or penicillin are common, if allergic to HCTZ.
- Increases calcium uptake by decreasing urinary calcium excretion and causing mild hypercalcemia.

- Can cause erectile dysfunction and photosensitivity (erythematous rash).
- Loss of serum sodium and potassium, mild pancreatitis, and mild metabolic alkalosis.

Contraindications:
- Gout, diabetes, renal disease, liver disease, hypokalemia, and hypotension.

Note: **Metolazone** is a thiazide-like medication.

β-blockers

Mechanism: Block the action of endogenous catecholamines.

Usage:
- Improves survival in patients with CHF and post-myocardial infarction.
  - Decreases heart rate, blood pressure and ejection fraction.
- Important anti-hypertensive medication that increases survival.
- Useful for cardiac arrhythmias, (atrial flutter, atrial fibrillation, sinus tachycardia, PVCs and PACs), CHF, glaucoma, mitral valve prolapse, HOCM, HCM, essential tremors, esophageal varices, acute hyperthyroidism, anxiety, and as prophylaxis for classic migraines.

Risk factors considerations of β-blockers:
- Sexual dysfunction and depression.
- Can exacerbated CHF if very low EF.
- Beware in patients with bradycardia, arrhythmia, hypotension, asthma, and COPD.

Overdose: IV calcium gluconate.

ACEIs

Mechanism: inhibits the angiotensin-converting enzyme.

Usage:

➤ *First-line treatment* for patients with diabetes, nephrotic syndrome, or congestive heart failure.

➤ Improves survival in post-MI and CHF patients.

Side effects:

▪ Dry cough, hyperkalemia, angioedema (only in about 0.1-0.7% of population), and renal failure in bilateral renal artery stenosis.

   • Angioedema is caused by bradykinin-mediated effects of ACEIs. The incidence is much lower with ARBs, such as **candesartan**.

   • Can cause dry cough because of increased kinin levels (switch to ARBs).

Note: **Losartan** can also cause angioedema.

Calcium-channel blockers

Usage: Isolated systolic hypertension, African-Americans resistant to β-blockers, Raynaud phenomenon (decreased vasospasm), Prinzmetal's angina, cerebral vasospasms, esophageal spasms, nutcracker esophagus, and elderly patients not tolerant of β-blockers.

Side effects: GI irritation, flushing, headaches, dizziness, and angioedema (in about 25% of patients after 6 months of use).

Note: diltiazem can cause peripheral symmetric edema.

Spironolactone

Mechanism: potassium sparing diuretic. Other potassium diuretics: **eplerenone**, **amiloride**, and **triamterene**.

Usage:

➤ Potassium-sparing diuretic; decreases mortality in patients with stage 3 or 4 congestive heart failure (has little effect on blood pressure).

➤ Used as aldosterone antagonist (primary hyperaldosteronism).

➤ Used to prevent hirsutism (in patients with PCOS and Cushing's syndrome).

- Used with other diuretics to prevent hypokalemia.
- Used to treat acne (anti-androgen effects).
- Shown to have mortality benefits in cases of systolic heart failure (helps inhibit aldosterone, which helps decrease fluid retention).

Adverse effects: gynecomastia (anti-androgen effects) and hyperkalemia (peaked T-waves).

Amiodarone

Usage: various types of arrhythmias, including ventricular tachycardia (if stable).

Side effects: PFTs, LFTs, and TFTs (pulmonary toxicity, liver toxicity, and thyroid toxicity).

- Thyroid function (TSH) should be tested every 4 months. Can develop hyper or hypothyroidism.
- If amiodarone is controlling arrhythmia well and patient develops hypothyroidism, recheck thyroid function in a few weeks or supplement with levothyroxine. Amiodarone decreases the conversion of T4 to T3, which increases T4 and decreases T3 levels.
- If pulmonary toxicity (interstitial lung disease) develops, withdraw medication.

Note: need to decrease warfarin dose by 25% after starting amiodarone.

α-1 receptor antagonist

Mechanism: α-adrenergic receptor antagonist.

Usage: Used for hypertension with or without BPH and helps with passage of kidney stones.

Side effects: Orthostatic hypotension (has a strong first dose response).

Clonidine

Mechanism of action: Stimulates α-2 adrenoceptors in the brain stem, which decreases PVR.

Usage:

- ➤ Short-acting sympathetic blocker acts on α-adrenergic stimulation; relieves hot flashes.
- ➤ ADHD, opioid withdrawal symptoms, and hypertension.

Risk factors: Abrupt cessation can cause rebound hypertension.

Note:

- ✓ Clonidine must be tapered.
- ✓ Other medications that need tapering are systemic steroids and phenytoin.

Atropine

Mechanism: an anti-cholinergic drug.

Usage: Bradycardia (*acute* symptoms) and organophosphates poisoning. Not commonly used to treat PEA or asystole, studies have shown it is not as beneficial, as once thought.

Side effects: Tachycardia, dizziness, AMS, dilated pupils, dry mouth, SVT, ventricular tachycardia, and ventricular fibrillation.

Dobutamine

Mechanism: Acts as a positive inotrope and decreases afterload, i.e., decreases the work against which the heart has to pump.

Usage: Treatment of acute CHF and cardiogenic shock.

Side effects: If a patient develops hypotension after dobutamine, **dopamine** can be given which has a positive pressor effect and increases afterload.

Nitroglycerin

Usage: stable angina, unstable angina, NSTEMI, STEMI, malignant hypertension, and pulmonary edema.

Side effects: *most common* side effect is headache. Orthostatic hypertension (is also a common feature).

Contraindications: use of α-1- blockers, right ventricular ischemia, HOCM, hypotension, or sildenafil.

Renal hypertension

Renal artery stenosis

Renal artery stenosis (narrowing of one or both renal arteries) leads to stimulation of the renin-angiotensin system, which leads to secondary hypertension.

➢ In case of middle-aged women, consider **fibromuscular dysplasia**.

➢ If aged >50 years, the cause is more likely to be atherosclerosis.

Hx/PE: Common clues are hypertension not controlled by medications and abdominal bruits. In case of abdominal bruits, consider both AAA and renal stenosis.

Diagnosis:
- *First*, evaluate urinalysis and BUN/Cr ratio.
- *First initial radiological study* is renal artery Doppler ultrasonography (*sensitive*).
- *Most accurate test*: renal angiogram (*specific*) but use with caution in case of renal failure (avoid contrast).

Treatment:
- Consider ACEIs in unilateral stenosis but never for bilateral stenosis.
- Optimal initial therapy is renal artery angioplasty with or without stenting.

Note: if marked increase in creatinine after initiation of ACEi therapy, this can lead to high suspicion of bilateral renal stenosis.

Pericardial diseases

Pericarditis

Inflammation of the pericardial tissue (tissue that covers the heart) which can lead to cardiac tamponade. Can be caused by infection (usually viral infection), idiopathic conditions, trauma, TB, SLE, uremia, drug use, radiation treatment, MI, or surgery.

Hx/PE: Fever, dyspnea, <u>sharp</u> chest pain (worsening with inspiration caused by friction rub), alleviation of pain with change in position. Worsening of pain when lying flat (stretch pericardium) and alleviation when sitting up and leaning forward.

<u>Physical examination:</u> triphasic friction rub/pericardial rub. Other common findings may or may not include increased JVD, hypotensive, and **pulsus paradoxus** (decreased systolic blood pressure of >10 mmHg with inspiration). **Kussmaul sign** (increased JVD on inhalation - should normally have decreased JVD on inhalation because the blood is pulled into the heart).

Diagnosis:

- *Optimal initial test* is EKG: ST-elevation in <u>all</u> leads (except aVR and V1) with PR segment depressions and sinus tachycardia. These are unique findings.

  - "**Electrical alternans**" may also be present but more common in pericardial tamponade.

- Troponin levels (to rule out MI).

- Chest radiography (to rule out pneumonia).

- Echocardiogram (to rule out tamponade).

- Consider ordering: CBC, electrolytes, ANA test, PPD, BUN/Cr ratio, uric acid, and UA.

Treatment: Treat underlying cause:

- NSAIDs (*treatment of choice*). SLE (corticosteroids/ immunosuppressant's). Uremia (dialysis). Post-MI (ASA).

Tamponade (pericardiocentesis). TB (antibiotics). Viral infection (NSAIDs/ASA).

- Steroids in *extreme* cases and addition of colchicine to increase efficacy of steroids.
- Surgery rarely needed.

Constrictive pericarditis

Results in a constrictive heart disease with fibrosis. Caused by chronic pericarditis, TB, viral infections, and others. Cardiac surgery or radiation history is a clue for constrictive pericarditis.

Hx/PE: Tachycardia, tachypnea, ascites, hepatomegaly, elevated JVD, "cardiac knock," and hypotension.

Diagnosis:

- EKG (low voltage), troponins, chest radiography (normal or calcification), and echocardiogram (decreased EF).
- Chest MRI (calcified and thick wall; *most specific test*).

Treatment: Diuretics, steroids, and *definitive treatment* is **pericardiectomy** (removal of the pericardium).

Note: with constrictive pericarditis, a pericardial knock can be heard in at least 50% of the patients.

Myocarditis

Inflammation of the actual heart muscle (myocardium). Mimics systolic heart failure because of damage to the heart tissue. Consequently, the heart cannot pump blood efficiently.

Diagnosis:

- ESR (elevated) and EKG (can present with arrhythmia or heart block).
- Troponins (elevated). Chest radiography (can be normal). Echocardiogram (low EF).
- Biopsy is the *most accurate test* (not usually performed).

Note: myocardial damage demonstrates elevated troponins.

Treatment:

- NSAIDs and glucocorticoids (to decrease inflammation).
- Treat symptomatic patients with medications for CHF (diuretics, ACEIs, β-blockers, low sodium, and low fluids).

Cardiac tamponade

Medical emergency

Fluid in the pericardial sac, compromised ventricular filling, and decreased cardiac output. Hypotension can cause death. Presence of 50 mL of fluid in the pericardium is considered normal.

Risk factors: the same factors that cause pericarditis can cause cardiac tamponade including, tuberculosis, trauma, myocardial ischemia, cardiac surgery, ventricle wall rupture, stab wounds, and aortic dissection.

Hx/PE: **Becks triad**: hypotension, JVD, and decreased heart sounds. Patient present with tachycardia and tachypnea. **Pulsus paradoxus** (decrease in systolic blood pressure >10 mmHg with normal inspiration). Need to rule out dehydration and pulmonary embolism; as can also present with hypotension.

Diagnosis:

- EKG: "**electrical alternans**" is the alternating of the height of the QRS complex (tall and short waves) and is practically diagnostic.
- Chest radiography (cardiomegaly).
- The *most accurate test* is echocardiogram: confirms diagnosis (decreased ejection fraction and fluid in the pericardial wall).
- Can perform a spiral CT scan (unnecessary in most cases).

Treatment:

- IV fluid expansion (also apply to right-sided infarct).
- Urgent **pericardiocentesis** (needle drainage), especially in unstable patient.
- In case of severe or long-term condition, **cardiac window** needs to be considered.

- If stable and secondary to uremic pericarditis, then consider dialysis.

- PEEP can be harmful because it increases intrathoracic pressure and decreases cardiac output.

Note: insert needle between the xiphoid process and the left costal margin in the direction of the left shoulder.

Valvular pathologies

Aortic stenosis

Calcified stenotic valve found *more common* in elderly populations, in which the most common presentation is chest pain (angina). Harsh systolic murmur best heard in the right second intercostal space (aortic area). Begins with LVH (S4 sound) and then progress to CHF (S3 sound) over time. Can have **paradoxical split** (pulmonary valve closing before the aortic valve). Systolic murmurs are heard when the blood flows forward. Associated with isolated systolic hypertension.

Hx/PE: Chest pain (*most common*), load S2, syncope, SOB, and "pulsus parvus et tardus" (weak and delayed pulses).

Classification:

➤ *Mild disease*: gradient across the valve, <25 mmHg.

➤ *Moderate disease*: 25-40 mmHg.

➤ Severe disease: >40 mmHg.

Diagnosis:

- EKG: LVH (left axis).

- *Optimal initial test*: echocardiogram (*most accurate*).

  - Transthoracic echocardiogram [TTE] *first*, followed by TEE, and catheterization (*last*).

- **Catheterization** is the *most accurate diagnostic test* for measuring pressure across the valve.

- Chest radiography (may show calcification).

Note: these steps are the same for all valvular diseases.

Review: valvular pathology must always *first* be determined with a non-invasive test such as TTE rather than invasive tests. If precise measurements are needed, use catheterization (*most accurate test* for measuring pressure).

Treatment:

- *Mild with hypertension:* ACEIs, ARBs, or calcium blockers to decrease afterload.
- *Severe:* balloon valvuloplasty is more useful in children with congenital stenosis or patients who are not eligible for surgery.
- Valve replacement is the treatment of choice for adults, as balloon valvuloplasty is not recommended.
  - Bioprosthetic valves: last about 10 years and warfarin is not required.
  - Mechanical valves: last about 15 years and warfarin is required.

Note:

✓ Do not use β-blockers in heart failure caused by aortic stenosis.

✓ Valvular angioplasty is more common in mitral stenosis (if asymptomatic) than in aortic stenosis.

Aortic regurgitation (AR)

"Early diastolic murmur" on the right second intercostal area, and decrescendo diastolic murmur (classic). Increased preload, increased end diastolic volume, and decreased ejection fraction. Diastolic murmurs are heard during retrograde blood flow.

Risk factors: ischemia is the *most common* risk factor. Our considerations are Marfan's syndrome, connective tissue disease, hypertension, CHF, endocarditis, aortic dissection, syphilis, ankylosing spondylitis, and rheumatic fever.

Hx/PE: All valvular heart diseases can involve shortness of breath (*most common* finding). Chronic AR can involve pulmonary congestion, dyspnea, orthopnea, Austin Flint, **Corrigan's pulse**, "water hammer pulse" (increase in pulse pressure), and Musset's sign (head bobbing up and down).

- ➤ Murmur increases with fist-clenching, squatting, and leg elevation.
- ➤ Murmur decreases with Valsalva maneuver and standing-up.

Diagnosis:

- EKG (left ventricular axis deviation).
- Chest radiography will show virtually the same findings in all valvular diseases.
- *Optimal initial test* is echocardiogram (diagnostic).
  - TTE followed by TEE.
- *Most accurate test* is catheterization.

Note:

- ✓ Intensity of murmurs of right-sided increases with inspiration (increased blood flow to the right side of heart)
- ✓ Intensity of murmurs of left-sided lesions increases with expiration (increased blood flow out of the heart).

Treatment:

- *First*, consider ACEIs, diuretics (furosemide), and digoxin.
  - All valvular heart diseases are associated with fluid overload, so diuretics are beneficial. However, diuretics are more beneficial for regurgitation than stenosis disease. Diuretics do not reverse the condition but slow the progression.
- Replace the valve surgically if ejection fraction is <50% (to avoid dilation of the walls).

Mitral valve stenosis

Most common etiological factor is rheumatic fever. Patients present with diastolic rumbling murmur with open snap, "**mid-late diastolic**"; heard best in the left 5th–6th intercostal space <u>midline</u>. Commonly associated with arrhythmias such as atrial fibrillation. Most common cause of death in 60% of the patients is CHF not arrhythmia. The left atrium is the most posterior structure of the heart and is located near the esophagus.

Hx/PE: Dysphagia (compressed esophagus), hoarseness (compressed laryngeal nerve), orthopnea, nocturnal dyspnea, arrhythmias, load S2, and enlarged left atrium.

➤ Murmurs increase with hand gripping, squatting, and expiration.

Diagnosis:

- These basic steps are the same for all valvular diseases:
  - Chest radiography (pleural effusions and left atrial enlargement).
  - EKG is not very helpful, as it only specifies where the hypertrophy is located.
  - The *optimal initial test* is echocardiogram (left atrium dilation). May also see RVH because of buildup of fluids. TTE (*sensitive*) followed by TEE (*specific*).
  - Catheterization (*most accurate test).*

Treatment:

- Diuretics and salt restriction (decrease fluid).
- **Balloon valvuloplasty** (with catheter) or mitral valve repair.
- Patients with mechanical valve replacement should be on both warfarin and aspirin.
- Administer warfarin in case of atrial fibrillation (keep INR between 2.0 and 3.0).
  - Control atrial fibrillation with β-blockers, verapamil, or digoxin.

Fun facts:

- If patient is *asymptomatic* <u>or</u> mitral valve area is >1.5 cm^2, perform a yearly follow-up with baseline EKG and repeat echocardiogram to evaluate stenosis progression.
- *Moderate/severe cases*: if the mitral valve area is <1.5 cm^2 or pulmonary artery pressure is >50 mmHg, then perform percutaneous balloon valvuloplasty.
- If balloon valvuloplasty is unsuccessful, valve replacement will be necessary.
- Percutaneous balloon valvuloplasty is the *most effective* therapy for mitral stenosis in pregnancy. However, valve replacement may be required after birth.
- Mother's health is always first priority.

Mitral valve regurgitation

Holosystolic/pansystolic murmur that radiates to the axilla or carotids. Resembles CHF with a murmur as a second finding. Regurgitation causes increased preload and end-diastolic volumes with decreased ejection fraction. Can be caused by damage to the chordae tendinea or by Ehlers-Danlos syndrome. Usually occurs after an MI.

Hx/PE: SOB, pulmonary edema, orthopnea, and nocturnal dyspnea.

➤ Murmur can be exacerbated with hand gripping and squatting (increased afterload).

➤ Valsalva maneuver and standing up (decreased afterload and decreased murmur).

Diagnosis: *Optimal initial test* is echocardiogram (TTE followed by TEE; will show regurgitant flow with increased left atrial and left ventricle size).

Treatment:

- Diuretics (ACEIs/ARBs) are the *best* medications.
- Digoxin might be useful.
- Valve replacement if *symptomatic*, and before the heart becomes dilated or EF reaches <60%.

Note: valve replacement criteria for mitral valve regurgitation is EF <60% and that for AR is EF <50%.

Mitral valve prolapse

Displacement of mitral valve into the LA during systolic contraction causing a "mid-to-late systolic murmur" at the apex (worsens with Valsalva maneuver and standing-up). Observed in about 2–5% of the population. *More common* among young women and those with Marfan's or Ehlers-Danlos syndrome.

Hx/PE: Usually asymptomatic or chest pain, palpitations, and panic attacks.

In mitral valve prolapse murmur sounds respond <u>opposite</u>:

➤ Standing-up and Valsalva maneuver: Increases the intensity of the murmurs.

➤ Hand gripping, leg elevation, and clenching fist: Decreases the intensity of the murmurs.

Diagnosis: Echocardiogram (*initial test*) and catheterization (*best test*) are rarely done.

Treatment:

- *Asymptomatic*: no treatment.
- *Symptomatic*: use β-blockers ([propranolol] for pain and panic attacks).
- Surgical repair is rarely needed.
- Endocarditis prophylaxis are not recommended.

Fun facts:

- For all murmurs (<u>except</u> for mitral valve prolapse and HOCM), hand gripping and squatting increase the intensity of murmurs (both these techniques increase forward blood flow).
- For all murmurs (<u>except</u> for mitral valve prolapse and HOCM), Valsalva maneuver and standing-up will decrease the intensity of the murmur (these techniques decrease forward blood flow).

  These are helpful techniques to distinguish the difference between mitral valve regurgitation and mitral valve prolapse.

- For treatment of mitral valve prolapse and HOCM, do <u>not</u> give diuretics but can use β-blockers. However, for all other valvular diseases, give diuretics and not β-blockers.

Pulmonary stenosis

Right ventricular hypertrophy and harsh systolic murmur in the left second to third interspaces (pulmonary area) with ejection click. Murmur radiates to the left and increases with inspiration.

Diagnosis: EKG (right axis), Chest radiography, EKG (right axis), and echocardiogram.

Treatment: Valve replacement or surgical repair.

Right sided murmur

Usually secondary to IV drug use. Usually a soft holosystolic murmur that increases with inspiration and heard in the left lower sternal border.

Thrombosis

Deep venous thrombosis (DVT)

Clots are more commonly formed in the deep veins of the lower extremities or pelvis.

Hx/PE: **Virchow's triad**: Venous stasis, endothelial trauma, and hypercoagulable states. Physical exam may show erythema, pain, and swelling in lower extremities. Positive **Homans' sign** (controversial) demonstrates lower extremity pain over calf on forceful dorsiflexion of the patient's foot, while knee is extended.

Diagnosis:

- Order: D-dimer levels (fibrin degradation product) and lower extremity Doppler scan (*sensitive*).
- If suspicion of <u>pulmonary embolism</u>: ABG, V/Q scan, CT angiogram (*specific*) or spiral CT scan (to confirm pulmonary embolism).

Note: refer to the pulmonology section of *In Your Pocket* for more details on pulmonary embolism.

Treatment:

- Unfractionated heparin <u>or</u> LMWH followed by warfarin (start after appropriately anticoagulated on heparin), or IVC filter (if medications contraindicated).
  - Before starting warfarin, assess hCG levels to rule out pregnancy (as this medication is teratogenic).

Note: no need to combined heparin and antiplatelet medications (aspirin).

Fun facts:

- While administrating warfarin, check PT/INR every day until the therapeutic range is reached for at least 2 days.

- While administrating heparin, check CBC (platelets) on day 3 and on day 5 to monitor for heparin-induced thrombocytopenia (HIT).

- HIT time frame:

  - Type I (1–4 days after administration): Usually non-immune-mediated disorder (no thrombosis or hemorrhage).

  - Type II (>5 days): Usually immune-mediated and heparin should be stopped (can lead to thrombosis).

    - Switch patient to argatroban or lepirudin.

Peripheral vascular disease

Peripheral arterial disease (PAD)

Occlusion of blood supply in the arteries by embolism or thrombus; more common in the lower extremities. Keep in mind that occlusions can cause compartment syndrome. It is important to control risk factors.

Risk factors: diabetes, hypertension, smoking, and hyperlipidemia.

➤ Acute ischemia: pain, pulselessness, pallor, poikilothermia, and paralysis.

➤ Chronic ischemia: complete lack of sensation can indicate irreversible state and may need amputation of extremity.

Hx/PE: Commonly relieved by rest (unless advanced). May also present with dorsal foot ulcerations and hairless, smooth, and shiny skin.

Diagnosis:

- *Best initial test*: Ankle-brachial index (ABI):

  - Range of 1.0 to 1.40 is normal.

  - 0.91 to 0.99 is considered borderline.

- <0.90 has a *specificity* of about 95% in indicating presence of the disease.
  - <0.40 indicates *severe* disease.
- ABI can decrease with exercise.
- Doppler ultrasonography (identify stenosis and occlusion).
- *Most accurate test* is CT angiogram (used for surgical evaluation).

Note: if patient is symptomatic with borderline/normal ABI, follow up with exercise ABI.

Treatment:

- *Long-term control*:
  - Control DM, HTN, and hyperlipidemia.
  - Exercise as tolerated, recommended 30 mins x 3 times a week (helps circulation).
- *Most single effective medication* is **cilostazol** (phospho-diesterase inhibitor), which is a direct arterial vasodilator that suppresses platelet aggregation and is indicated for medical management of peripheral claudication along with exercise.
- If medications are ineffective (including aspirin, statins, clopidogrel, and dipyridamole), then
- revascularization can be considered.
  - Angioplasty and stenting (*gold standard*).
  - Arterial bypass and amputation (*last resort*).

Note:

✓ Avoid non-selective β-blockers because they can cause peripheral vasoconstriction.

✓ Selective B1 blockers are <u>not</u> contraindicated.

✓ Cilostazol is contraindicated in heart failure.

Steel pulse syndrome

This may occur when the *subclavian artery* is occluded proximal to the origin of the vertebral artery.

Hx/PE: Pain in the upper extremities, coldness, and tingling *more commonly* induced with exercise.

Diagnosis:

- *Best initial step* is to compare blood pressure in both upper extremities.
  - If systolic blood pressure difference is >15 mmHg, perform duplex ultrasonography *followed* by CT or MRI angiography.

Treatment: Angioplasty, stenting, bypass, or amputation.

Lymphedema

Lymphedema

Disruption of *lymphatic circulation* causing peripheral edema and chronic infection.

<u>Risk factors</u>: surgical procedures involving lymph node dissection.

Hx/PE: An example would be post-mastectomy with swelling in the upper extremity. Physical exam reveals peripheral edema, erythema, and tenderness.

Diagnosis: Rule out: DVTs, cardiac disorders, cirrhosis, and nephrotic syndrome (transudative processes). Be vigilant of cellulitis.

Treatment: Compression garments, exercise, and massage can be helpful.

Note: diuretics are not effective with lymphedema.

Syncope

Syncope

Temporary loss of consciousness and postural tone caused by cerebral hypoperfusion, which usually lasts <30 seconds. Commonly of cardiac origin but can be of non-cardiac origin.

Causes:

➤ **Cardiac syncope**: arrhythmias, hypotension, valvular disease, pulmonary embolism, and aortic dissection. Usually short-lived and associated with a history of cardiac abnormalities.

➤ **Non-cardiac syncope**: orthostatic hypotension, hypovolemia, stroke, seizure, TIA, vasovagal response, and metabolic abnormalities.

Hx/PE: Light headedness, dizziness, muffled sounds, pallor, and weakness.

Diagnosis:

- Orders will depend on suspicion: CBC, electrolytes, ABG, glucose, TSH, EKG, troponins, echocardiogram, 24-hour Holter monitoring, orthostatics, brain MRI, and EEG.

  - **Tilt-table test** (decrease systolic blood pressure >20 mmHg or decrease diastolic blood pressure >10 mmHg).

- Vasovagal syncope is a clinical diagnosis and no further tests are needed. Unless uncertain use upright tilt table testing.

Treatment: Etiology based need to treat the underlying cause.

Cardiology Index

Symbols

α-1 receptor antagonist 44
β-blockers 42

A

abdominal aortic aneurysm 34
ACEIs 42
adenosine 9
amiloride 43
amiodarone 44
angina 19
angioplasty 32
aortic abdominal aneurysm 34
aortic dissection 35
aortic regurgitation 51
aortic stenosis 50
asystole 10
atrial fibrillation 4
atrial flutter 5
atrioventricular block 2
atropine 45

B

balloon valvuloplasty 53
Becks triad 49
blue toe syndrome 33

C

CABG 32
calcium-channel blockers 43
candesartan 43
cardiac syncope 60
cardiac tamponade 49
cardiac window 49
catheterization 50
CHADS score 11
chest pain, common causes 24
cilostazol 58
clonidine 45
complete heart block 3
constrictive pericarditis 48

coronary angiogram 32
coronary artery bypass grafting 32
coronary artery disease 18
Corrigan's pulse 51

D

deep venous thrombosis 56
diastolic dysfunction 15
digoxin-binding antibody 17
dilated cardiomyopathy 14
dobutamine 45
dopamine 45
Dressler's syndrome 25

E

endomyocardial biopsy 18
eplerenone 43
essential hypertension 37
exercise stress test 32
exercise thallium test 33

F

fibromuscular dysplasia. 46

H

hydrochlorothiazide 41
hypercholesterolemia 36
hypertension 37
hypertensive emergency 40
hypertensive encephalopathy 39
hypertensive urgency 39
hypertrophic cardiomyopathy 16
hypertrophic obstructive cardiomy-
      opathy 16

I

ischemic heart disease 18
isolated systolic hypertension 39,
      50

Index, cont'd

K

Kerley B lines 14

L

LBBB 29
left circumflex coronary artery 29
losartan 43
lymphedema 59

M

malignant hypertension 40
maximal stress test 34
metolazone 42
mitral valve prolapse 54
mitral valve regurgitation 54
mitral valve stenosis 52
Mobitz type I block 3
Mobitz type II block 3
multifocal atrial tachycardia 5
myocardial infarction 22
myocarditis 48
myomectomy 17

N

nitroglycerin 46
non-cardiac syncope 60
non-ST-elevation myocardial in-
        farction 22
NSTEMI 22
NYHA = CHF 11

O

OCP-related hypertension 41
ompartment syndrome 57

P

paradoxical split 29, 50
pericardiectomy 48
pericardiocentesis 49
pericarditis 47
peripheral arterial disease 57

prehypertension 38
premature atrial contractions 6
premature ventricular contractions
        6
Primary HOCM 16
Prinzmetal's angina 21
procainamide 10
pulmonary stenosis 55
pulseless electrical activity 10
pulseless ventricular tachycardia 7
P-wave 29

Q

QRS wave 29

R

RBBB 29
renal artery stenosis 46
renal hypertension 46
restrictive cardiomyopathy 17
right sided murmur 56

S

Secondary (HCM) 16
secondary hypertension 39
second-degree block 3
sinus bradycardia 1
sinus tachycardia 1
spironolactone 43
stable angina 19
stage 1 hypertension 38
stage 2 hypertension 38
steel pulse syndrom 58
ST-elevation myocardial infarction
        23
STEMI 23
stress test 32
submaximal stress test 33
supraventricular tachycardia 9
syncope 60
systolic dysfunction 12

Index, cont'd

T

thallium test 33
third-degree block 3
thoracic aortic aneurysm 34
thrombosis 56
torsades de pointes 8
triamterene 43
T wave 29

U

unstable angina 20

V

ventricular fibrillation 8
ventricular tachycardia 7
Virchow's triad 56

W

Wenckebach block 3
Wolf-Parkinson-White syndrome 9

X

xanthelasmas 36
xanthomas: 36

www.ingramcontent.com/pod-product-compliance
Lightning Source LLC
Chambersburg PA
CBHW040839180526
45159CB00001B/242